Dedication

This book is dedicated to my mother, Olie Pearl Grant, who taught me the meaning of true love. I would also like to acknowledge my father and brother, Harry Hall Grant and Tyrone Grant, whom I love and miss dearly. Last, but certainly not least, I must also mention Virginia D. Perry, the matriarch who started it all. May they continue to rock the heavens and be my guardian angels.

Table of Contents

Preface

My journey to becoming a CRNA was long and untraditional. I want to share it with you so that your journey can hopefully be smoother than mine was. My purpose is to give you the information and resources necessary to be where you want to be sooner than later. I did not have mentors to guide me and the answers to my questions were not easily accessible at the time I pursued this career. I wrote this book to not only assist you in your own journey, but to also instill in you the motivation and inspiration you may need to finally take the leap of faith.

Aside from a lack of guidance, the beginning stages of my adult life were filled with many ups and downs. I am telling you my story because I know that if I can do it, so can you. We all go through trials and tribulations, but it's what you do to overcome them that will determine your future.

Do I have all of the answers? Absolutely, not. I am still growing, learning, and advancing in my own path. However, the knowledge that I've acquired over the last twenty years will help you achieve your dreams and desires in a more efficient way. If my story can help one person do one thing better than the way that I did it, then my work is done.

I hope you enjoy this book and that it not only answers your questions, but also gives you the encouragement and energy to pursue *your* dreams like I did. Whether you want to be a CRNA, RN, NP, any other type of medical professional, or not, I hope and pray that this serves you well. While reading about my journey you will learn that nothing was granted to me quickly or easily except my last name.

Introduction

The 90s was by far one of my favorite decades. I grew up in western Massachusetts with my parents and three much older brothers – nine, thirteen, and eighteen years older to be exact. I absolutely loved everything about that place and time, from the music to the clothing. Come to think of it, there was only one thing that I never enjoyed – the cold weather. Six months of dark cold gray skies and snow was not something I enjoyed. For that reason, I decided early on that I was going to either UNC Chapel Hill or Georgetown for college. Aside from the weather, my decision was rooted in the simple fact that I liked their basketball team colors.

No one in my family had attended a four-year university, but my mother told me from a young age that I was definitely going to college. To be what? I had no idea. I thought about becoming a lawyer, but I learned in high school that I really disliked arguing. Plus, I was too shy to stand up and speak publicly, so that wasn't going to work. I was always a good student growing up, partly because my mother wouldn't have it any other way. So, there were a lot of avenues I could have chosen, but at that time I hadn't really put too much thought into it. Regardless of what my career path was going to be, my mother taught me that I always needed to be able to take care of myself and to never rely on anyone else to provide for me financially. It was ironic because I was very spoiled by her growing up, and no one thought I'd ever survive on my own. The love and support she had for me was like nothing I've ever experienced again in my lifetime. She was my biggest advocate, supporter, and cheerleader.

My career path was somewhat chosen for me in 1996 when I was sixteen and my mother signed me up for a certified nursing assistant (CNA) course. She was a licensed practical nurse (LPN) and worked two jobs from as early as I can remember. My mother knew that as a CNA I could work as much or as little as I wanted to, as well as get a first-hand view of what was done in the nursing field.

I worked as a CNA off and on throughout high school and college, making an hourly wage of $7 to $10. That was *big* money for me back then, especially compared to my first job at RAVE clothing store for $4.15 an hour. I enjoyed working part-time during high school because I was able to cash my checks and go shopping on my days off. I had a savings account that very rarely had much more than a hundred dollars in it at any given time, because I knew that if I ever needed more money, I could always just ask my mother.

When I started working as a CNA, I was also attending a brand new public high school, which I transferred to in eleventh grade. I was part of the first graduating class of the High School of Science and Technology in Springfield, Massachusetts. Although this was a different environment for me – I transferred from a Catholic school that I had attended from fifth to tenth grades – I absolutely loved the last two years of my high school experience and often reminisce about how great those times were. One of the fondest memories I have from high school is a trip to Spain I took during senior year with my Spanish class. My mother joined us as a chaperone, and for the second time in her life, traveled outside of the United States. We had an amazing time there and one day planned on returning.

By the spring of 1998 I had been accepted to all of the colleges my mother and I vetted and decided would be best for me. After deliberating together, it was determined that I was going to attend Campbell University in Buies Creek, North Carolina, majoring in Biology with a pre-physician assistant concentration.

Campbell had a five-year physician assistant program, and even though I visited the school during spring break, I still chose to go there. You'll know why I say that if you've ever been to Buies Creek. To paint the picture for you, there was only one flashing stop light and, if you were hungry, you had either a Subway restaurant or Pizza Hut to choose from. This was all located in the neighboring town about four miles away from the college campus, which had just as much character. The closest large city was an hour away.

One month after we returned from that trip to Spain I mentioned earlier, and two weeks after I graduated high school, my mother was diagnosed with stage IV uterine cancer. Two weeks after that diagnosis, she woke up one morning and could no longer see. She had developed a retinal tear and was determined to be legally blind. From that day on, she could no longer work and our world was flipped upside down within a four-week period. My father was retired from his city job and received a small pension, but there weren't many other sources of income for my family. Although this was thrown at us all at once, and I wanted to stay by her side, my mother insisted I not change my college plans. I'm not really sure why I didn't focus more on applying to colleges closer to home once that news had been shared. Looking back, I really feel like it's because I didn't have much guidance; at the age of eighteen, I did not understand the death sentence that had been handed to my mom.

So, with apprehension, I moved down to Buies Creek that summer for my freshman year. Although it was ultimately my decision to go, I wasn't completely sold on the major or the college I had chosen; I was just going through the motions. I was preoccupied thinking about my mother going through chemo and radiation therapies after having a total hysterectomy just a couple of months earlier. As a teenager, I really had no grasp on what any of this meant, but I just did the best I could to make my parents proud. For the most part, I did well in my classes, but I was very unhappy being down there, in the middle of nowhere, with my mother five hundred miles away slowly dying.

As soon as freshman year ended, I begged my mother to let me transfer to another university. Against her better judgment, she told me that I could, but made it clear that she was not supportive of my decision. I applied and was accepted into North Carolina A&T State University in Greensboro, which is an HBCU (historically black colleges and universities). I *immediately* felt at home there even though I was still 500 miles away from my home in Massachusetts.

There was no physician assistant program there, so I decided on nursing. I knew that as a nurse I could always find a job and be able to take care of myself financially. It was in that nursing program where I learned about the profession of certified registered nurse anesthetist (CRNA). My interest was piqued because CRNAs have a lot of autonomy and, more importantly, a high salary range. That day in 1999, as I sat in Noble Hall, I decided right then and there that I was going to be a CRNA.

In September 2000, as I began my junior year of nursing school, my mother passed away at the age of fifty-nine; I was twenty-years-old. I still remember today, over eighteen years later, picking up the phone that early morning and hearing that she died overnight in the North Carolina home of my brother, Tyrone. He had taken care of her those last few months of her life. I remember crying in the bed as my sister-in-law broke the news to me. After that, I never liked hearing the phone ring early in the morning again.

The same day that my mother passed away, I had a big medical-surgical exam that I could not miss. I knew that my classmates could tell something was wrong. I sat down, finished the exam, and left. Somehow, with everything going on, I got a 94%. Failing out of school was not an option, especially since I now had to provide for myself. My mother instilled in me enough of her strength and passion that I knew it was time to be independent, even if I didn't necessarily know how.

I graduated *summa cum laude* in May 2002 and had secured a job in the medical intensive care unit (MICU) at Rex Hospital in Raleigh, North Carolina. I studied for the NCLEX-RN exam (National Council Licensure Examination for Registered Nurse) the entire time I was in nursing school, so I felt confident and set my test date right after graduation. I drove to Virginia to take the exam because all of the testing dates in North Carolina were booked, and I needed to take it before my MICU externship start date. There was no way I was going to mess that up; they were going to pay me $17.10, a $3 evening shift differential, and a $5 weekend differential, all by the hour. No one could tell me anything at that point. I knew I was going to be doing *big* things, and that was an understatement. Little did I know...but we will get back to that.

When I took the NCLEX-RN, the computer turned off after I answered eighty questions. I didn't know what that meant, so I was left anxious and wondering. I called every day for one week straight to hear whether or not I had passed – back then, you didn't get your results immediately. Finally, one day about a week after taking the test, I called and the automated machine read me my new RN license number. I passed! I was now a registered nurse.

Attending nursing school and working as an RN in the MICU were two very different things, more so than I had imagined. Since I went to an HBCU school, I was used to seeing "melanated" professional faces all around me. It was a very empowering environment to be in. However, in the ICU at Rex, that was not the case. There wasn't much diversity, and I was one of only two black nurses in the unit. The long hours also threw me for a loop. I worked twelve-hour night shifts and ended up gaining twenty-five pounds. I also became very moody and depressed. As you can imagine, losing my mother at such a young age had a great impact on me. Although I was sticking to "the plan," I was left feeling lost and alone, like I didn't fit in anywhere or with anyone. I was five hundred miles away from my closest family members, trying to figure out the ways of life all on my own. Also, my shyness kept me in the house on most of my days off.

Through all of this, I still thought about going to CRNA school and took a GRE (Graduate Record Examination) prep course that was offered by the hospital. I studied using flash cards in my spare time and on my days off. I took the GRE a year after I graduated from nursing school and scored fairly average with 700/1000 – the scoring system is different now than it was back then.

I began talking myself out of applying to CRNA programs around that time because I was convinced that I wasn't ready and that I didn't have enough experience. So, I began travel nursing instead. I took assignments mostly within the Northeast of the United States and really started to enjoy being a nurse. Of course, the paychecks didn't hurt either. With my salary as a traveling nurse now being double what it was as a staff nurse, I was able to pay off loans from undergraduate school. After two years of working as a registered nurse, I decided to apply to a nurse practitioner program and take courses online. I actually liked being a student and really missed the feel of the college experience, although online courses weren't the same as campus courses. Nevertheless, I still enjoyed the learning aspect. So, I ended up taking three graduate level courses, nursing theory, pharmacology and a research class, finishing with a 4.0 GPA.

I continued working as a traveling nurse and enjoying my life, taking trips to other countries. I even took assignments around the holidays in order to be closer to my family members in New England. I also purchased a Lexus, my dream car. At the age of twenty-four my credit score was the best it has ever been, given I had every credit card imaginable and a car note. Looking from the outside, you could say I was definitely "living the good life." In actuality, I was totally misguided and had nothing tangible to show for all of the work I was doing and the money I was making. On top of that, I felt unfulfilled because I still wasn't living out my dream of becoming a CRNA. Like I said, superficially I was winning, but the next six years would be filled with many hills and valleys, so my dream was put on hold.

In 2006, I received another daunting phone call. My father was sick and dying from cancer. I learned that while he was in Connecticut visiting a distant relative, he woke up extremely ill one morning, was rushed to the hospital in Massachusetts, and diagnosed with stage IV pancreatic cancer. Apparently, he'd known about it for a few years but told none of us. He spent the remaining months of his life at Tyrone's home in North Carolina, just like my mother had done.

I'll give you the abridged version of the roller coaster ride my life was on for those six years. At one point, I got engaged and moved to Florida only to break it off and return to North Carolina. I made new "friends," who would later become strangers, but also gained a new best friend. I began riding motorcycles and purchased a Kawasaki Ninja 600 which became my newest toy. In 2007, I also purchased a brand-new home because, well, that's what everyone else around me was doing. I moved out of my free travel nursing apartment into my beautiful new townhome. As luck would have it, the recession hit in 2008, and the travel nursing market dried up. Most companies were now offering a salary close to what I was making as a new graduate six years prior, and there were barely any assignments to choose from. Even regular nursing jobs were scarce and more difficult to find.

I do, however, remember a high point during this rocky time. One night, while at one of the *per diem* jobs I had, a couple I worked with – I have now forgotten their names – told me that I was too young and too smart not to be a CRNA, and that I just needed to do it. "But wasn't I too old now?" I thought. I definitely felt too old at that point to go back to school. In January 2009, Barack Obama was inaugurated as President of the United States. Politics aside, when I saw that man and his family on stage, it lit a fire underneath me. I decided it was finally time for me to pursue the dream that I had originally set out for seven years prior.

Then, another low happened. That summer of 2009, while I was applying to CRNA school and going on interviews, I got one of those dreadful early morning phone calls again. This time, just one week after his forty-first birthday, I was told that my older brother, Tyrone, had been killed instantly in a motorcycle accident on his way home from work after a long night shift. I was in shock. Just days prior to his accident, we spoke about riding our motorcycles together, which is something we bonded over. When Tyrone was taking care of my mother and father during their last few months of life, he and I grew closer from my weekly visits. He and his wife would often have me over on the weekends and during the holidays. Tyrone was very supportive of me pursuing CRNA school. I've only ridden my motorcycle once since his death.

To make matters worse, at the time of my brother's passing I was in a very emotionally abusive and toxic relationship with a man that was manipulative and narcissistic. Unfortunately, I learned that the hard way. I stayed with him because I felt like he was all I had, and I kept hoping that things would return back to the way they were when we first met. This was a very dark period of time for me, mentally and financially, as the economy was deep into the recession and I was let go from my full-time nursing job. If I didn't get accepted into a CRNA program soon, I was going to think about removing myself from the clinical aspects of nursing all together.

I finally left that tumultuous relationship, and I'm so glad I did. It was during one of the lowest points in my life that I finally managed to get my "YES". I had applied to seven different programs, went on five interviews, and was waitlisted by one prior to getting accepted on the sixth try. It was two days after the break up that I received an email from the program director at the former University of Medicine and Dentistry of New Jersey (UMDNJ), now Rutgers University-Newark, asking whether or not I was going to accept their offer. Apparently, they mailed the acceptance letter to my home in North Carolina weeks prior while I was working in Massachusetts, but my ex never told me about it. The most important thing I learned at that point in my life is that not everyone can go with you where God is trying to take you. Once you close one door the Universe can, and will, open up so many others.

Over the course of that nine-year period with tremendous highs and lows, I learned that the craziest part about losing someone whom you love dearly is that life continues on even when you feel like you can't. Therefore being proactive in healing from loss and pain is something that you must accomplish on your own, for the most part. I took the next several years of my life to not only heal from the traumas loss had brought me, but also to learn more about who I was and how I could learn to love myself without needing someone else. You are responsible for your happiness and no one can fully fill a void in your life except you. Though I am still a work in progress, I can now look back and see just how much I've grown over the past eighteen years.

Chapter 1: What is a CRNA?

A CRNA (certified registered nurse anesthetist or anesthesiologist) is an advanced practice registered nurse who holds a graduate or doctoral degree with a concentration in anesthesia. For the purpose of this book I will use the term CRNA to mean nurse anesthetist or nurse anesthesiologist. Nurse anesthesiologist was termed a reasonable designation for all CRNAs by the American Association of Nurse Anesthetists in 2018. Nurse anesthetists currently provide and administer over 45,000,000 anesthetics each year in hospitals, surgical centers, eye centers, endoscopy suites, dentist offices, and many more locations. The practice began over one hundred years ago in the Civil War era with the first nurse anesthetist by the name of Alice Magaw. She began practicing in 1893 with Dr. Charles Mayo and his wife. The actual CRNA credential came into existence in 1956.

The AANA's Scope of Nurse Anesthesia Practice reflects that CRNAs are licensed, independent practitioners who provide comprehensive anesthesia services. CRNAs are not an extension of physicians, nor are they dependent on physicians to provide anesthesia services. CRNAs practice both autonomously and in collaboration with other healthcare professionals on an inter-professional team to deliver high-quality, holistic, patient-centered, and evidence-based anesthesia and pain care services. Nurse anesthetists care for patients of all acuity levels across the lifespan of the patient in a variety of settings for procedures including, but not limited to, surgical, obstetrical, diagnostic, therapeutic, and pain management. CRNAs also serve in leadership roles in healthcare delivery organizations.

CRNAs are a vital part of the health care team. In some states CRNAs and physician anesthesiologists may work together as a

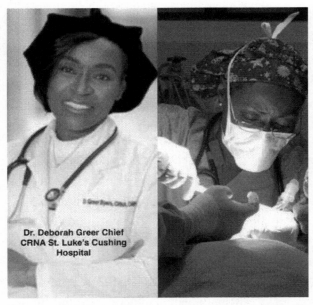

Dr. Deborah Greer Chief CRNA St. Luke's Cushing Hospital

team or the nurse anesthetist may work independently. Currently nurse anesthetists are the main anesthesia providers in most rural areas and to the men and women of the U.S. armed forces. According to U.S. News and World Report, the career is one of the top-rated medical professions in the United States with a job growth rate of about 16% over the next ten years and an overall career satisfaction score of 7.9 out of 10.

As a certified registered nurse anesthetist, I am with the patient before, during, and after the operative procedure. I bring them to the operating room, help position them onto the table, place monitoring devices on them and get them ready "to go to sleep." I administer the drugs to induce them into unconsciousness, place breathing devices in their airway, maintain a therapeutic level of anesthesia during surgery, and wake them up when it's over. I make sure patients are not experiencing pain, nausea, or vomiting when I drop them off in the post-anesthesia care unit. Unless given a break at some point during surgery, I'm always caring for the patient while he or she is under anesthesia. I work in collaboration with physician anesthesiologists at my current facility.

Chapter 2: What Type of People Become CRNAs?

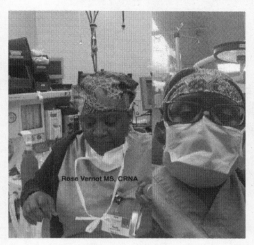

Rose Vernot MS, CRNA

To answer the question of the type of person who generally becomes a CRNA, I asked Dr. Thomas Pallaria, DNP, CRNA, APN. Dr. Pallaria is the Program Director and Regional Chief CRNA of the Department of Anesthesiology at St. Barnabas/Newark Beth Israel/Overlook Medical Center. According to him, "The ideal SRNA candidate will be in the top 5% academically, will have practiced for a minimum of two to three years in the highest acuity critical care area, and be able to demonstrate through written and verbal communication a commitment to lifelong learning." I would like to add that CRNAs are well-organized, usually have Type A personalities, are confident, and are able to manage working with different personalities. CRNAs have great time management and organizational skills, are effective communicators, and enjoy scientific learning.

Chapter 3: How Do I Become a CRNA?

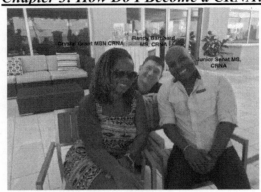

Degree Requirements. In order to meet the application requirements for a CRNA program, you must hold a bachelor's degree in nursing (BSN). Alternately, a Bachelor of Science degree in chemistry, physics, or biology *and* an associate degree in nursing is required. You can also hold an MSN (Master of Science degree in nursing) with a different concentration and apply. Note that by 2022 all nurse anesthesiology programs will be doctoral level. That is the DNP (Doctor of Nursing Practice) and DNAP (Doctor of Nurse Anesthesia Practice), either varying in length from thirty-one to fifty months of study. CRNAs are now graduating with doctoral degrees and have studied research concepts and aspects in the anesthesia communities.

If you have obtained your associate degree, you can begin working in the intensive care unit as an RN while going back to school for your BSN, either online or on campus. There's more than one way to get to the finish line; what's important is that you start the process. For CRNA school, undergraduate college courses in inorganic and organic chemistry, anatomy and physiology, microbiology, and statistics will be required. These courses must be taken within ten years of submitting your application, with at least a

B grade. A final GPA of 3.0 or higher in your last sixty months of undergraduate coursework is considered competitive. Official, sealed transcripts of all undergraduate and graduate level courses taken will also be required.

ICU Experience. One full working year of ICU experience is the minimum amount that CRNA programs require, but at least two years' experience is preferred. Your RN license needs to remain clean and untarnished, so there cannot be any negative occurrences pending on it. A minimum of 2,000 full-time hours of ICU work prior to the start of a program is recommended. That's not to say that you can't also be working on the other necessary application requirements at the same time, such as taking the GRE (Graduate Record Exam), which is required for some programs.

GRE. The GRE is basically the SAT (Scholastic Assessment Test) of graduate school. There are three graded parts to it: quantitative reasoning, verbal reasoning, and analytical writing. The scores range between 130-170 for the quantitative and verbal sections, with a total score of 300 being considered competitive in most programs. A 3.5 or greater on the analytical writing section is also desirable on a scale ranging from 0-6. Don't fret if your total score is lower. You can retake the GRE up to five times within a calendar year and choose which scores you want sent with your admissions application. Currently, the fee is $205 for the GRE, and scores are valid for five years.

Letters of Recommendation. Three letters of recommendation will be required for most program applications. Each letter should be from someone who can attest to your strengths and knowledge as an ICU nurse, such as your unit manager, charge nurse, an educator, a surgeon, or another doctor with whom you have a close working relationship. I suggest asking several different people in order to have more than the required amount of reference letters. That way, if you plan on applying to multiple schools you

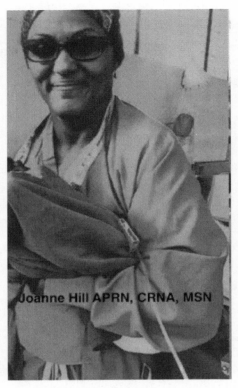

Joanne Hill APRN, CRNA, MSN

don't have to keep asking the same people to write your reference letters. These references are key to the application process, so make sure you choose people you know will write a strong statement about your strengths as a potential student. Also, thoroughly read the application requirements on the website for each program. They may want letters of recommendation from specific sources and submitted in a particular way.

Shadowing Experience. It is strongly advised, if not absolutely necessary, that you shadow a CRNA. Shadowing means closely observing and following a CRNA throughout their day. You will do this once you are already an RN as most hospitals have strict criteria for allowing unauthorized personnel into the sterile operating room. Some schools have a verification form that the CRNA you shadowed must fill out.

Finding one to shadow may be a tad difficult, but if you're working in the ICU, you may have direct access to meeting a CRNA who brings the patients to you after surgery. When I worked in the CTICU (cardiothoracic intensive care unit), the CRNAs who did the anesthesia for heart surgeries were the ones who also brought the patients to me from the operating room and who gave me the reports. Working nights can make that a challenge depending on where it is you work. However, it's more than likely that your colleagues will be trying to get into school as well, and they may know a CRNA who you can shadow. You can also contact someone in the anesthesia department at your facility and ask to speak to the chief CRNA to request and schedule a date to shadow.

Letter of Intent or Personal Statement. You will need to write a letter of intent or personal statement. This letter is essentially telling the program why they should pick you. So, why should they pick you? Here are some examples of what your statement could include: What have you done to make yourself stand out as an applicant? Do you volunteer? Are you a charge nurse or preceptor in your unit? How many times have you shadowed a CRNA? Do you teach ACLS (Advanced Cardiac Life Support), PALS (Pediatric Advanced Life Support), or BLS (Basic Life Support)? Are you a flight, trauma, or army nurse? Is your name known in the nursing or anesthesia community? Have you contacted the program director? Have you shadowed the chief CRNA at the hospital affiliated with the program? Are you on the code or rapid response team? Have you been a paramedic or firefighter before? Is this your first or second career? What is your passion, and how has it brought you to apply to this program? Did a special patient or family member open your eyes to this career? Have you been to a diversity CRNA event?

When writing your letter of intent or personal statement, you need to think about what is going to set you apart from the hundreds of other applicants applying to the program. Make sure you "cross all the t's and dot all the i's" on your application paperwork. Edit, spell check and then edit some more. Put that Type A personality into overdrive when writing your letter and let who you are shine through your words.

Certifications. It is imperative to complete courses in BLS, ACLS, and PALS as these certifications are required to work in the ICU. In the courses, you will learn about the drugs that are given during "codes" which indicate different emergency situations. You will also learn more about 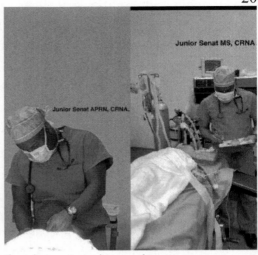 EKG (electrocardiogram) rhythm interpretation and treatments.

Curriculum Vitae. Your curriculum vitae (CV), which is similar to a résumé, will also be part of your application package. If you need assistance with preparing one, there are many résumé builders and other online resources that can be of assistance.

CCRN Exam. The CCRN is a certification exam given by the AACN (American Association of Critical-Care Nurses). Passing the exam indicates that you have met the knowledge requirements to care for patients in an acute or critical care setting. The test is comprised of 150 questions, including twenty-five practice questions, and a minimum score of 87% is needed in order to pass. Currently, the cost for the exam is $340 if you are not a member of AACN and $235 for members. The annual AACN membership fee is $78 and the certification is valid for three years.

In order to sit for the exam you have to meet certain criteria when it comes to your working hours. The AACN website specifies that you can either "practice as an RN or APRN for 1,750 hours in direct care of acutely/critically ill adult patients during the previous two years, with 875 of those hours accrued in the most recent year preceding application *or* practice as an RN or APRN for at least five years with a minimum of 2,000 hours in direct care of acutely/critically ill adult patients, with 144 of those hours accrued in the most recent year preceding application."

I asked one DNP SRNA – the 'S' in SRNA stands for 'student' – about her thoughts on the exam. She shared, "Not only is the CCRN helpful to get into anesthesia school, it is a respected credential to have in the workplace. I found practice questions to be the best preparation, as they reinforced the content and question formats. Laura Gasparis Vonfrolio has a highly recommended

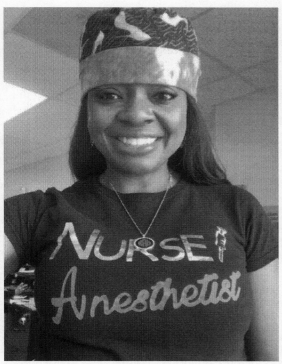

review course. Many hospitals provide an incentive to RNs who obtain advanced certification. It is an exciting accomplishment and I recommend it to all critical care nurses."

Application Fee. The application fee, which differs by school, should be sent in with all of the other required paperwork. Make sure you submit all application materials prior to the deadline. These schools receive so many applications, and sometimes make admissions decisions early. If you send your application on or close to the deadline, it could be too late and there may not be a space for you. Every school has a different application deadline and program start date. If you're planning to apply to more than one program, I recommend using a spreadsheet to stay organized and help you keep track of admissions deadlines and all of the required materials for each program.

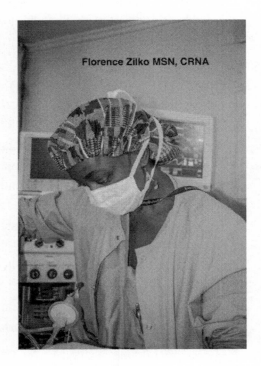

Florence Zilko MSN, CRNA

Chapter 4: How Much Does CRNA School Cost?

Currently, there is a wide range of program costs anywhere from free all the way up to and beyond $200,000. If you are accepted into a public program in the state that you reside in, you don't have to pay out-of-state tuition and fees. It is likely that during the interview process you will be asked about your family's financial situation, because it is strongly suggested that you do not work while in the program due to its intensity and time commitment. You may be thinking, "So, how do I pay for school?" Well, ideally, you've planned for this ahead of time and have saved quite a bit of cash to pay for school.

I say that, because I should have saved up instead of buying new cars, a new house, and going on trips. I had absolutely no money saved after eight years of working as an RN because I spent it all. As a result, I ended up taking out over $125,000 in student loans in order to pay for my graduate education and living expenses. I did that because I didn't know any better and had no guidance on the matter. No one ever taught me about living below your means to save money, so I spent everything I made. Although I watched Suze Orman on television and read her books for years, I really don't remember her speaking about living debt free and saving money. She spoke more about having a good credit score and retirement plans, both of which I had in my twenties while working as a nurse. So, by the time I graduated, the interest on my student loan accrued and I owed close to $200,000. Luckily, I have a career that allows me to comfortably manage my payments.

I paid for the mistakes I made in my twenties once I became a CRNA in my mid-thirties. Speaking from experience, my recommendation is to save as much money as you possibly can once you secure your first job after nursing school. You can reward

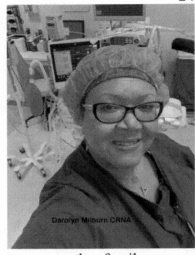

yourself with something nice every once in a while, but saving should be a priority to properly prepare for the financial commitment of a CRNA program. To save even more, take extra shifts while you're working in the ICU and put all of that extra money away. Live like you're still a broke college student even when you're working over forty hours per week as an RN. You can also get a second or third job if overtime isn't available in your hospital. If you have parents or other family members that will let you live with them, then do that. The amount of money and stress you will save yourself is unimaginable. Look at it this way, once you graduate and start working, you'll be able to repay your loved ones with an all-expenses-paid cruise to the Bahamas as a thank you for their kindness and generosity. That first CRNA paycheck is going to be all yours to enjoy; trust me, it'll be a big one.

If saving way ahead of time is not an option for you, like in my case, consider joining the armed forces. That way some of your tuition will be covered in return for time served upon graduation. Definitely do your research on the requirements for joining the armed forces. You can call and speak to a recruiter to obtain more information.

There are some anesthesia groups and hospitals that will pay a stipend to students who work for them. This amount can range anywhere from a couple hundred dollars a month to the entire cost of tuition. If you go that route, you will be indebted to the group or facility upon graduation for a certain amount of time, so make sure you know all of the details before signing on the dotted line.

Scholarships and grants are also available. If you've received support this way during your undergraduate studies, then you should be familiar with the process. Sometimes your school will have information about scholarships and grants, and someone will suggest that you apply for them. If not, you will have to spend time researching online. Essays and letters of recommendation are usually required for scholarships and grants, but the time and effort is well worth receiving "free" money to further your education.

Of course, the last option is taking out student loans. If you received student loans for college, then you should know the process. In case you aren't familiar, there is an online form called the FAFSA (Free Application for Federal Student Aid) that you will fill out for graduate school. The application requires your previous year's tax return, and a PIN that they assign you, in addition to other documents. The purpose is to find out which loans and/or grants you are eligible for. In order to receive funds, you will have to sign a loan promissory note once the school year begins. It is important to note that Grad Plus Loans may need to be acquired in order to supplement the remaining cost that the government loans may not cover. With a grad plus loan you need to have a good credit history. Adverse events on your credit such as foreclosure, bankruptcy or repossession will make you ineligible to receive them. The use of a cosigner may also be needed if your credit isn't good enough. Other than FAFSA, you can look into private bank loans and credit cards to pay for some tuition and fees. The interest rates may be higher or lower than the government-funded loans depending on a number of factors, including your credit score. While I am not a financial advisor, my personal opinion about using credit cards is to avoid doing so unless absolutely necessary.

I'll give you an example of what I was doing with credit, and hopefully you won't make the same mistakes. I would use the money from my student loan to cover room and board. Whatever I had leftover was for the rest of my living expenses for that semester. I also had two credit cards with pretty high limits that were close to being maxed out.

Six months prior to the end of my program, I ran out of money. I was still paying for a house in North Carolina – even though I had tenants, they're rent payments did not cover everything – on top of a car payment, insurance, gas, and food. I am grateful that one of my classmates was kind enough to loan me money so that I could make it through the last six months of my program. Had she not helped me out, I honestly

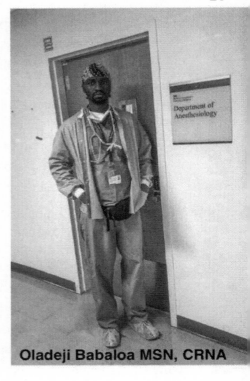

Oladeji Babaloa MSN, CRNA

don't know what I would've done. I had no source of income over the past two years, so getting a private loan wasn't an option. Also, I was single, so there was no supplemental income. Only with the help from my classmate was I able to make it financially *almost* to the end of the program.

With a little over four weeks left before graduation, we were hit by hurricane Sandy. Newark was hit pretty hard and we were without power for almost a week. I applied for a credit increase; since I was in an area that had been devastated by the hurricane, they granted the increase. I'm not saying I was happy to have that hurricane hit us so hard, but I am grateful that I was able to benefit financially, allowing me to make it through to the end of the program. The very last thing I did after graduating was took out a payday loan. I do not recommend doing this unless absolutely necessary. The interest rates on these alone are enough to give you angina.

Chapter 5: I Got an Interview!

Congratulations! You have ICU experience, took your GRE, shadowed a CRNA, submitted your application, and received an email or letter asking you to come in for an interview. After your initial excitement subsides, you will reply to the invitation either accepting or declining. Why would you decline an interview? There may be personal reasons, or you may have already been accepted to your school of choice; turning down an interview is okay.

For the interview, dress clean and professionally and, of course, show up early. Different programs have varying interview protocols. For some, you might meet one-on-one with the program director. For others, you may sit in front of a panel of several interviewers. Interviewing can be very nerve-racking, and so is being a CRNA at times, so preparation is key. In order to be confident and secure, I recommend becoming familiar with common interview questions and practicing your answers. Clinical questions are

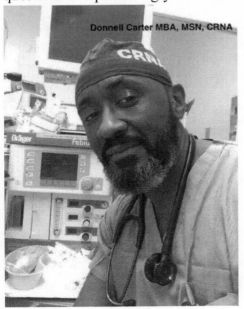

Donnell Carter MBA, MSN, CRNA

popular, so make sure you feel comfortable answering specific questions about the type of ICU patients you've worked with. Also, if you will have to relocate to attend the program, they may ask if you are prepared for that. Overall, the interviewers want to know that you will be a good fit for their intensive program and that they will be a good fit for you. You should also prepare for your interviews by visiting the AANA and your state nurse anesthesia association websites to research current topics of interest in anesthesia. Some schools may do a practical interview where you are put in a mock clinical situation and asked to provide care for a patient. Always be yourself, be confident, and take action. You've got this!

After the interview, you will eventually hear back from the program either way. Once wait listed or accepted, you have to send in a monetary deposit in order to hold your spot. If you are waitlisted, don't look at it as a bad thing; it just means that your application is being held and you could likely get a spot if one opens up. People change their mind and life happens. Keep interviewing and be prepared for a possible last-minute call that you've been accepted into a class that starts in a month.

Take it from Dr. Tedrick Vernon, DNP, CRNA and his experience. He shared, "I applied and interviewed at Duke University's program and was waitlisted. Despite everyone telling me it was still possible to get in, I began feeling as though I wasn't good enough. I eventually came out of my self-pity and told myself that if I was good enough for Duke's waitlist then I know for a fact I can get in at another school. I chose five additional schools and gave myself one year to make it happen. I also looked at my finances and expenses. I did everything that I could to displace being waitlisted. I even began preparing applications for the next [admissions cycle] so I could be one of the first to get mine submitted. Low and behold, three months later when I least expected it, I got a call back from Duke telling me I was in. Being waitlisted had no bearing on my success. I graduated with a 3.9 GPA and won the award for clinical excellence."

Chapter 6: What About My Family?

A tremendous amount of time and commitment is necessary to get through CRNA school. Your time management and organizational skills will quickly be put to test between studying for exams, preparing for clinical, working on projects, and still trying to keep your sanity. Your family may not understand the amount of time you're going to need in order to study and excel as a student.

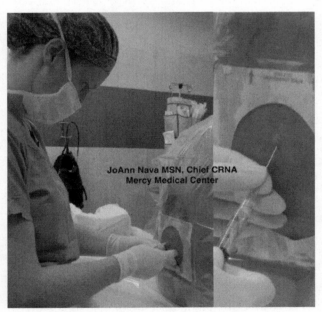
JoAnn Nava MSN, Chief CRNA
Mercy Medical Center

Therefore, they may feel neglected, or resentful, once you're actually in school. It's extremely important to have the conversation with them beforehand about what it's going to take and how you're going to need their love and support. This will have to be a team effort between you and your spouse, or any other family members with you during the process, for the next three years; it will all be worth it in the end.

A married couple I know suggest that if you have problems in your marriage or relationship before-hand, you should attempt to settle those issues before beginning the program. The commitment required for the program will likely put a further strain on things.

Explain the sacrifice you are making in order to be happier as well as to support the family financially once you become a CRNA. You will need your spouse to hold down the fort for the duration of your time in school. Although I don't have statistics on the matter, I know there are correlations between attending CRNA school and divorce and infidelity. Don't let this scare you if you're in a relationship, but do talk about it with your significant other beforehand. Just because some people experienced this hardship, it doesn't mean that it will happen with your relationship, but it's good to be aware.

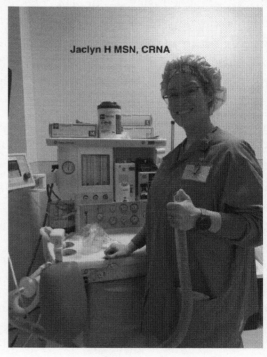

Jaclyn H MSN, CRNA

Chapter 7: What is CRNA School Like?

Classes will include anatomy and physiology, pharmacology, health assessment, biochemistry, pathophysiology, anesthesia physiology, obstetrics, regional anesthesia, pediatric anesthesia, physics and chemistry. Aside from classes, it's important to supplement your learning with additional reading and studying in order to grasp all of the information. Search the internet for helpful weblinks and YouTube videos on topics that are difficult to understand.

Tests in each subject are usually given anywhere from once a week to once a month. There will also be group and individual presentations on various topics. You'll be taking more than one course at a time so, as I mentioned before, good time management is imperative when it comes to studying for different exams on multiple subjects. Exams are computerized and timed in order to prepare you for taking the "anesthesia boards", the NCE (National Certification Examination for Licensure and Certification).

Clinical rotations in a number of departments are a major part of CRNA school. These include general surgery, pediatrics, obstetrics, cardiac, trauma, and regional/pain management. A clinical preceptor, either a nurse anesthetist or physician anesthesiologist, may supervise you depending on the clinical site. You will learn how to administer epidurals and spinal blocks to pregnant women and manage their well-being throughout the delivery. You'll also learn how to place central lines and arterial lines for an entire coronary artery bypass on a patient who has heart or vascular disease. You will learn anesthesia for a wide range of cases, from taking care of children who need tubes put in their ears to managing an elderly patient undergoing a hip replacement. You will sedate patients having a colonoscopy, eye surgery, or even having a bunion repaired. Your clinical schedule may fluctuate between eight, ten, sixteen, and twenty-four-hour shifts. When you graduate, you will have over 2,500 clinical hours on top of the clinical hours you put in as an ICU nurse.

Depending on your program, you may have to be on call overnight. This could result in tending to emergency situations in the middle of the night, such as having to administer anesthesia to a trauma victim with a gunshot wound or do an emergency C-section at 3 a.m. You will be shown how to perform different regional anesthesia blocks like femoral, axillary, and bier. Basically, you will see a lot and get to do a lot throughout this part of the program. You're also going to be working with many different anesthesia providers, so be sure to soak up as much knowledge and skill as possible.

Don't be surprised if you have to go to clinical on holidays and weekends. However, some programs do make accommodations for religious observations. On the other hand, there are programs that do not have clinical on nights, holidays, and weekends. Make sure you do the necessary research on the program you wish to attend if clinical schedules may be an issue for you.

There are two types of CRNA programs. The first type is called front-loaded. This means that you take all of your coursework in your first year of the program. The second half of a front-loaded program is in the clinical setting. This is where you will put everything that you learned from the prior year in the classroom to use in the operating room. The other type of program is called integrated. Unlike front-loaded, in an integrated program you complete coursework and go to clinical together the entire time, taking courses that coincide with the clinical setting you are in or will be in. If one type of program sounds better to you than the other, make sure you apply to the programs that fit your learning needs.

Thomasina Frimpong LeClair, MS, CRNA, APRN shared her experience: "During clinicals I still had classes. They were once to twice a week in the beginning with three to four clinical days. Gradually, we went to once a month by the time we were in the OR (operating room) alone. We only had a preceptor for the first three to three and a half months. When the seniors graduated, we all were in the OR by ourselves, with an attending anesthesiologist 2:1. That ratio means that the anesthesiologist was watching over two rooms while the SRNAs were in the rooms doing the work."

Another colleague, a DNP SRNA who prefers to stay anonymous, stated, "There are pros and cons to front-loaded and integrated programs. I appreciate the opportunity to have hands on experience that parallels what is covered in class; it makes the

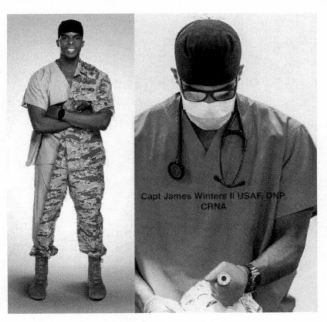

Capt James Winters II USAF, DNP CRNA

information more tangible. On the other hand, it is not uncommon to have a knowledge gap between what is covered in class and clinical, thus it is the student's responsibility to be proactive and research cases and conditions in depth and prepare for what may happen. Even with preparation, unexpected scenarios and questions will present. Be upfront and inform the preceptor you have not yet covered the concept due to the structure of your program. Be humble, eager to learn, and pursue the information at a later time. Both paths get you to the same great destination. Choose the program that fits your personality, lifestyle, and budget. You can't go wrong!"

Attending one to three state conferences may also be required of your program in order to learn the political side of a career in anesthesia. A benefit of joining the AANA as a student is getting to observe more about the politics as well as network with others in the profession.

A certain amount of sick or vacation days are usually allotted to use throughout the entire length of the program. When considering time off, keep in mind that you must hit all of your clinical hours and numbers on certain skills. If you're out too much and don't reach the quota, you may have to make up missed days at the end of the program.

Chapter 8: I Finished School. Now What?

I made it all the way to graduation and moved back to Massachusetts, which was where I had signed on to take my first CRNA job. I lived with my niece and her husband because I had no money and nowhere else to go at the time. I still had to take the NCE and began studying for it shortly after I moved back home.

The previous summer, I took a review course by Valley Anesthesia. I studied for six weeks straight, from 7 a.m. to 7 p.m., Monday through Saturday. I reviewed all of the information that I learned over and over again to the point where very simple things that I knew well started to confuse me. It was at that time that I knew I had to take the boards. I paid the fee and scheduled a test date. Some of my other classmates had already taken the test and passed, so I was feeling good.

One cold January morning, I went to the testing center and went through all of the standardized testing motions. I sat at my computer and began the exam. The first ten questions were so difficult that I hoped they were practice questions. When question eleven came, I thought I had sat down for the wrong exam. I began to panic, which I normally don't do. I'm not a nervous test taker at all, but I had so much riding on passing this exam. I didn't have another $800 to retake it should I fail. I literally had $600 in my bank account, and I was weeks away from beginning work and receiving my first paycheck. Plus, I already had a start date for my new job and didn't know if that could be changed. I was sleeping in my five-year-old great niece's bed and desperately needed my own space once I could afford to move.

Midway through the test, I broke down and began crying. In that moment, I prayed to God and my mother in heaven to give me the strength and knowledge I needed in order to continue. I looked

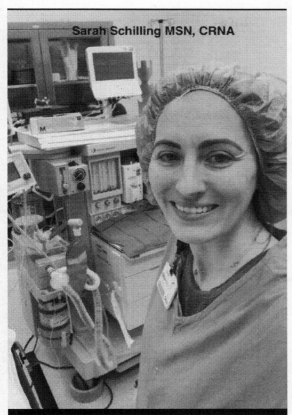
Sarah Schilling MSN, CRNA

down at the computer timer and saw time ticking away. Unfortunately, the timer doesn't stop just because you're having a mental breakdown. Somehow, from deep inside of me, I found the strength that I needed and picked my head back up. I told myself that I knew this information and that I was prepared to answer these questions. I began going through the test again, this time much more level-headed and clear-minded. All of a sudden, about thirty minutes later, the computer shut off. I gasped because I thought I had done something wrong. I remembered being told in my review prep class, "if the computer is on, then you're still in the game." However, if it turns off after a certain amount of questions, you either did so poorly that there's no chance of passing *or* you successfully answered enough questions to show competency. Although I was unsure about a lot of the questions, I didn't think that I had done so poorly to cause the algorithm to give up on me and turn off the computer. I got up from my seat and went out to the proctor, who smiled and handed me a paper with "PASS" on it. I burst into tears and asked if I could hug her – she said yes, by the way.

Chapter 9: What Happens After I Graduate?

Finally, the day has arrived. You have completed all of your didactic coursework, clocked in 2,500 clinical hours at various medical facilities, and your Doctoral Capstone has been submitted and approved. You've studied for hours, taken the NCE, and passed, meeting the requirements of the NBCRNA (National Board of Certification & Recertification of Nurse Anesthetists). So, now what do you do? You might want to take a vacation to celebrate your achievement or buy yourself a fancy new car or house with those new checks coming in soon. Before we get carried away, let's take a few breaths and think some things through, like where you're going to work. Hopefully you have already applied, interviewed, and received a formal job offer before graduating. That is the ideal way to transition from school to work with no gap in between. I had a job lined up one year before I finished school.

As far as the types of facilities you can work in, there are anesthesia groups owned by anesthesiologists or CRNAs. Alternately, you may work as a hospital employee or even freelance as an independent contractor. In large teaching hospitals, anesthesiology residents will usually be given first dibs on larger cases because they also need to learn anesthesia. You will get them as well, but certain procedures like heart surgeries, neurosurgeries, epidurals, and other regional techniques will go to them first. If you really want to be involved in those types of cases, make sure you mention that in your interview and to the person who makes out the daily schedule. Speaking up about wanting to be on larger cases will notify the scheduler to add you onto the list of providers who want to do them. Note that not all large teaching hospitals have an anesthesiology residency program, so you may very well do the anesthesia for all of those large cases. Additionally, there may be a large amount of operating rooms, which means greater availability of large cases.

Community hospitals are another option for where to work. These smaller facilities generally do not take on large trauma cases, which are usually routed to a trauma center. Some may do vascular, neurological, spine, or lung cases. CRNAs are the number one providers in rural areas and may be the sole anesthesia provider in such a setting, providing all anesthetics to a wide range of patient populations. Whether you're in a large teaching hospital or small community hospital is entirely up to you and your comfort level.

There is also a large need for CRNAs in a number of settings outside of the hospital, including eye centers, endoscopy centers, dental offices, plastic surgery centers, and day surgery centers, to name a few. In choosing the right workplace for you, make sure you are comfortable with the salary, benefits, and scheduling. It's also a good idea to speak to another CRNA, besides the chief, who already works at the facility to find out the scoop. Before signing any contract, know and understand what you are agreeing to; make sure that is the right place for you. There is a plethora of job openings; I get emails, texts, and phone calls almost daily for CRNA positions. The job market is hot, so don't settle just because the offer seems good at the time, and always negotiate if the numbers are too low for you. The worst that can happen is that they say no. Also be wary and informed about groups that offer sign on bonuses for a certain amount of time commitment. Once you accept that money you are locked in with them for the given time period. If you take the job and end up not liking it or needing to move prior to your contract being fulfilled they are going to want their money back from you sometimes with interest. Another catch with that is the money that they give to you is taxed, but if you have to repay them you need to repay the entire amount not the taxed amount you received.

If you haven't already guessed by now, once I graduated I spent my first few paychecks reimbursing my classmate who lent me money while I was in school. A few months after that, I moved out of my niece's house, and into my own apartment, and started working on my DNP online. I took out even more student loans to do that.

The following year, I got married and paid cash for the wedding and honeymoon. I also bought a beautiful silver on black BMW four series and became a dog mom of two. One day, my now ex-husband and I were talking and trying to figure out where all of our money was going. We had nothing to show for it and we were living paycheck to paycheck. I realized I had adopted my old spending habits from my twenties because I still didn't know any better. I began listening to Dave Ramsey in March 2016 and we implemented a financial plan that day. With a little more than $350,000 in debt, he and I began the debt-snowball method. Upon writing this, I have paid off over $254,000 of my debt with only my student loans left. Had I started on those when I first graduated in 2012, they would be long gone by now, but such is life. I look forward to the day – my goal is by end of 2020 – I can do my debt free scream and be so much happier financially than I have ever been. Although most of my money still belongs to Great Lakes, I have a clearer financial picture of how to win with money. I'm not telling you that you

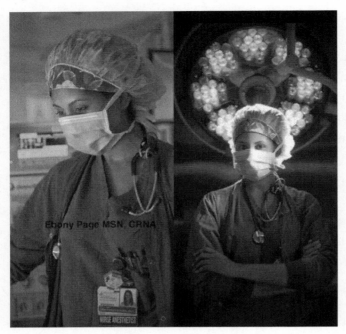

Ebony Page MSN, CRNA

shouldn't buy yourself a big house or fancy car after you've worked so hard, but I am urging you to be smart about it. So, sit down and crunch the numbers first to see what your financial situation would look like if you took the two to three years to eliminate your debts and then began saving huge chunks of your very high salary to buy assets in cash instead of making payments with interest on liabilities.

Chapter 10: Paperwork, Paperwork, and More Paperwork

The day you pass your CRNA board exam is not going to be the day you begin working as a CRNA. There is a process called credentialing that needs to take place prior to you beginning at your facility. The process of credentialing can begin while you're close to graduating and have accepted a position. However, the final documents needed to complete credentialing are available after you finish the program and pass the boards. A copy of your degree, malpractice insurance history, RN license, NBCRNA card after passing boards, driver's license, PALS/ACLS/BLS certifications, as well as letters of reference are just some of the required documentation. For each facility you work in, credentialing paperwork will need to be done first. This is because there isn't a registered agency that keeps all CRNA information in one place for credentialing purposes. Credentialing can take anywhere from two weeks to six months depending on the facility and how quickly you submit the required paperwork.

Depending on the state you live in, you will usually have to renew your RN and CRNA license every two years. Most employers will reimburse you for that cost. Recertification of ACLS, PALS, and BLS is required, and may also be reimbursed by the group you work for. If you work full-time as a freelancer, then paying for work items is a business expense that can be deducted from your taxes. The NBCRNA requires a certain amount of continuing education credits over a four-year span, specifically, twenty-five credits per year broken up into class A and class B. Currently there is a two-year check in period required during the four-year cycle and cost $110. If you elect to be a member of the AANA after you graduate, then that cost is $645 every year which may be reimbursed by your employer.

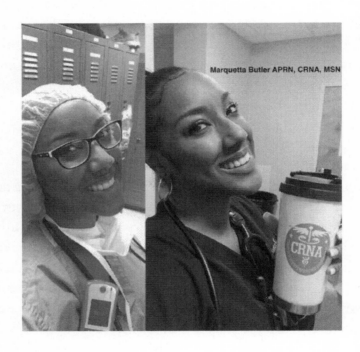

Marquetta Butler APRN, CRNA, MSN

FAQs

I have received many questions from individuals curious about becoming a CRNA, and I decided to share them with you along with my answers. Some of the answers contain a lot of jargon that you may not be familiar with if you do not work in the medical field, but that's okay, and I encourage you to do further research on anything you are unsure or curious about. You can also contact me with any questions you have (see *About the Author* page). Keep in mind that responses are based on my experience, my observations, conversations with colleagues, and my own research.

Q: What do you love most about being a CRNA?
A: I love working with one patient at a time and giving them my undivided attention. I love being there for each patient at a very vulnerable time in his or her life, because even the "smallest" procedure or operation can be a "big deal" and anxiety-provoking. I love the comfort I can bring to them with the techniques that I am skilled and mastered in. I also enjoy the freedom my career affords me and the lifestyle I am able to live. I love learning new techniques from my anesthesia colleagues as there is not only one way to beautifully administer an anesthetic.

Q: Is CRNA school hard?
A: The program is challenging and definitely requires commitment, as described in chapter seven. There is a massive amount of information you will be taught and need to know. The classes are graduate level courses. There is a lot of information crammed into a small amount of time. Self-directed learning and studying, about forty hours a week, will be necessary outside of class in order to be successful. The number of hours will vary depending on how

quickly you are able to understand and retain the information. There is also a capstone project that is required for your doctorate.

Q: How difficult is clinical?
A: The first few times you go to clinical, it will more than likely be for eight-hour days. You won't know what's going on, where to stand, what to touch or where to go. You will learn everything from where to find your scrubs to where to put your lunch. Your locker combination or badge may not work, and no one will be there to help. You won't know how your preceptor likes the room set up, but you'll do an outstanding anesthesia machine check. Every single thing you do, even if it seems insignificant, is part of the learning process. Each day, you'll have a new preceptor who likes his or her room set up differently, and you'll be doing different anesthetics for various procedures. I also recommend factoring in time to prepare for clinical and being there early to set up your room to see patients. Some schools require that you create a care plan and present it to your preceptor for each surgery you participate in. If you're lucky, your clinical site will be close to where you live; otherwise, you may have to travel up to an hour or more. So, waking up at 3 a.m. to get ready and hit the road isn't unheard of. All of this will take time to master; then boom! At the end of that rotation, you'll be sent to another clinical site for the next rotation to start the process all over again. I can reassure you that it does get better and, with time, many tasks will become easier and like second nature. Don't get discouraged and definitely don't give up. We've all been there.

Q: Is it cold in the operating room?
A: The AORN (Association of periOperative Registered Nurses) recommends the temperature in the operating room to be between sixty-eight and seventy-two degrees Fahrenheit. Sometimes the

surgical team gets warm and requests the temperature be decreased. If you're usually cold, I advise layering up.

Q: How do I pay for school?
A: Chapter three is all about ways to pay for CRNA school. Saving money and paying your tuition in cash is the ideal method that I recommend. Scholarships, grants, and loans are also available if you do the research and find them. Stipends from anesthesia groups in exchange for a work commitment and joining the armed forces are also options. Working is usually not advised during these programs, so make sure you have a financial plan in place before you start.

Q: Should I take out loans for school?
A: Yes, but only if you absolutely have to. Use your savings, apply for grants and scholarships, ask different anesthesia groups if they will pay for your schooling with an agreement that you work for them after graduating. If all else fails, take out loans. I talk more about this in chapter four.

Q: Why are you so against student loans?
A: I am not against student loans so much as I am against using loans improperly and without a plan, like I did. I didn't know much about finances when I took out loans and, even while working with a financial planner once I became a CRNA, I saw very little of my paychecks going anywhere. I purchased a new BMW – leased it actually – paid for a wedding, and took vacations often. In 2016, I adopted the teachings of Mr. Dave Ramsey and have been able to pay off over $235,000 since working his plan. I encourage those around me to also adopt his plan to pay off debt, especially if you are young and can take advantage of compounding interest. It took me thirty-six years to learn how to make my money work for me instead of the other way around.

Q: Am I too old to go to CRNA school?
A: The average age of a CRNA student is twenty-nine, but don't let age deter you if you are much younger or older. It's never too late.

Q: Should I get married before, during, or after school?
A: That's an extremely personal decision, but I think it depends on how much assistance you have with planning, paying for, and executing your wedding vision. If you decide to get married while attending CRNA school, just know that you may have a limited number of days off approved for the wedding and honeymoon. The time commitment for planning a wedding will also be limited due to school obligations and, of course, your budget may be greatly impacted by the cost of tuition. Speak to your significant other and decide on what will work best for the two of you. Keep in mind that a wedding doesn't have to be big and expensive; you can get married at the courthouse with a Justice of the Peace.

Q: Should I have a child while I'm in school?
A: If you're a female of childbearing age and desire to get pregnant at a certain time in life then I strongly suggest speaking to your spouse and/or other family members about this. You will need assistance since you won't be granted much time off to have a baby once you're in a program. Leaving the program and returning the following year may be an option that you would have to speak to your program director about. If you already have children, then enlisting the help of family and friends may be crucial. A colleague of mine, Jillian Cullinane, MSN, CRNA, APRN states, "As a mother of a nine-month-old and a six-year-old, I relied heavily on the help and support of my husband and parents. Nurse anesthesia training was one of the most stressful and challenging experiences I have ever been through. To succeed, I needed to be very organized, and as

hard as it was, pull myself away from family and events to study alone. It wasn't easy, but with intense discipline, time management, and hard work I achieved my goal of graduating from CRNA school."

Q: What if I got bad grades in college?

A: If you made some poor choices as an undergrad, or just had a difficult time learning the information, I suggest retaking the courses you did poorly in. If you want to apply to CRNA school and it's been longer than ten years since you completed the required coursework, you will have to retake them. Try your hardest to get an A in each of those courses the second time around. That will show the admissions committee that you know you made mistakes in the past and now you're doing what is needed to improve. You can also take the graduate entry-level courses, and must call the school beforehand to inquire about the courses that can be taken prior to being accepted into a program. Also, work your hardest to get A's in those classes to prove once again that you're serious about furthering your education.

Q: What if I don't get accepted into a program?

A: If you've applied to more than one program and were declined from one, then you are still in the game as you await notice from the others. If you were not granted an interview then I would suggest calling the program that did not accept you to ask what you can do differently, and better, for next years' application process. If you were granted an interview and it didn't go well, then practice your answers to common interview questions (see next question) with someone else for the following year. Applying to more than one program will obviously increase your odds of getting an acceptance letter. I applied to seven, interviewed for five, was waitlisted for one, and got accepted into one. All you need is one YES.

Q: What are some examples of CRNA school interview questions I might be asked?
A: In no particular order, here is a list of many questions that interviewers will ask, as well as some probing statements. Note that this list is not exhaustive, so there may be other questions you get asked that are not shown here.

- What extracurricular activities are you involved in?

- What was the last journal article you read?

- Tell me about your nursing experience.

- Why do you want to become a CRNA?

- Tell us what steps you have taken to prepare for this program financially, academically, professionally, and personally.

- How do you handle stress?

- In a group setting, what role do you play?

- If a colleague asked you to waste a narcotic but had already discarded the syringe, what would you do?

- Walk me through the pathophysiology of septic shock.

Here are some common written interview questions:

- The monitor goes flatline during a case. What is the first thing you would do?

- How do you float a swan ganz catheter?

- What is renal dose dopamine?

- List 3 cases of postoperative tachycardia.

- List 3 interventions for a patient having crushing chest pain radiating to the jaw.

- List interventions for a patient with high pressure limiting on the ventilator.

- List ACLS interventions including doses.

- Calculate a dobutamine drip in mcg/kg/min.

- Interpret a sample ABG (arterial blood gas test).

- Write an essay on JCAHO's (Joint Commission on Accreditation of Healthcare Organizations) safe patient standards and how that relates to your current practice.

- How would you describe yourself?

- How would your manager describe you?

- What are your strengths? What are your weaknesses?

- Give an example of a recent conflict you encountered and how you dealt with it.

- Tell us your short-term goals.

- What are your long-term goals?

- What will you do if you are not accepted into our program?

Q: What were your study habits?
A: My program was an integrated one. The first semester I took three courses and studied every day after class and on the weekends. I went to weekly study sessions with a small group of classmates, and we would go over the information for hours until it finally made sense. We began clinical one day a week in our second semester and

attended class during the rest of the week. The next semester, over the summer, we went to clinical two days per week and had class twice a week. I studied whenever I wasn't in class or preparing for clinical. Time management is crucial during a program. If you have children and other family obligations then you will have to manage your time wisely.

Q: Will I be prepared to take CRNA boards?
A: The short answer is yes. After all of your experience in the ICU, over three years of anesthesia school, and 9,000 hours of total clinical experience, you have been groomed to be successful. If you want to prepare further, there are review courses you can pay for and attend given by a number of businesses. The two I know of are Apex Anesthesia and Valley Anesthesia Review – I am not endorsing either program. As of January 2019, the boards cost $995 to take and you will need proof of graduation from your program director prior to setting a test date. The test is given in all fifty states in English only. It is computerized and timed.

Q: What happens if I fail my boards?
A: If you fail the board exam, the NBCRNA will send you an assessment of the areas that you scored low. Focus on studying those elements and schedule your retest date. You will have to repay the fee of $995. You can retake the exam four times within one calendar year for two consecutive years. After eight unsuccessful attempts you will be required to re-enroll in another accredited CRNA program.

Q: Isn't nursing for women only?
A: Definitely not. Actually, 40% of CRNAs are men. If you are a male and considering the nursing profession, know that your population in the field will only continue to increase.

Q: What nationalities are represented in the CRNA profession?
A: From a 2016 survey, the ethnic breakdown of 53,000 CRNAs and SRNAs is as follows: 1% African American, 2% Hispanic, 3% Pacific Islander, 0% Native American, 4% other/non-Caucasian, and 90% White/Caucasian. For more information about diversity visit diversitycrna.org or https://www.aana.com/about-us/aana-diversity-and-inclusion.

Q: I heard that CRNAs get sued a lot. Is that true?
A: I can't speak to the frequency of lawsuits against CRNAs, but I do know that any profession in the medical field comes with high liability. As a nurse anesthetist you will have malpractice insurance coverage provided by your anesthesia group and you can also purchase additional coverage on your own through a private company or through the AANA. If you are going to be self-employed and receive a 1099 tax form, then you will need to purchase your own malpractice coverage. Some agencies will provide it for you and others will offer it on a per shift basis in which they deduct a few dollars per hour from each paycheck. There are two types of insurance policies: occurrence and claims made. Should a lawsuit arise, your medical malpractice insurance will kick in. Most policies cover you from $1M to $3M. The statute of limitations is also different in each state, so the amount of time someone has to sue following an incident varies.

Q: How much money do CRNAs make and how much time off do they get?
A: A full-time CRNA salary varies by state and employer. The current national median is $160,250 per year. Overtime and on-call time may or may not be factored into that amount. Usually, you get paid more if you work more, but sometimes the salary remains the same regardless of your daily or weekly hours. A total compensation package can include sick time, holidays, vacation time, health and retirement benefits, and profit sharing in addition to your base salary. I know of CRNAs who are millionaires; they either own their own businesses or increase their wealth through sources of passive income. It can be done. Paid time off can range anywhere from four to twenty-six weeks – yes, there are positions out there that offer so much time off, usually alternating weeks with another CRNA in a rural setting. Short-term and long-term disability may also be a benefit offered. That means you will still get paid if you are injured and can't work for an extended period of time. Usually, disability insurance covers 60% of your salary. If you or your partner have a baby, you can use your short-term disability during maternity/paternity leave. As an independent contractor, you can save up enough money to stay afloat and take as much time off as you'd like with your newborn or for any other reason.

Q: What kind of jobs do CRNAs work?
A: CRNAs can work in a variety of settings. See chapter nine for more details.

Q: What kind of ICU should I work in?
A: One to two years of experience in a level one trauma hospital is essential. CVICU (cardiovascular), CTICU (cardiothoracic), STICU (surgical trauma), TICU (trauma), and transplant ICU are, in my opinion, the top intensive care units that I suggest you get experience

in. Learn as much as possible and become proficient within your unit. I highly recommend gaining knowledge of the following: ventilator modes and settings, EKG interpretation, intra-aortic balloon pump, ECMO (extracorporeal membrane oxygenation), dialysis, ABG analysis, Swan-Ganz catheter, and vasopressor intravenous (IV) drips. The level of acuity of these patients will give you a large advantage and the basic knowledge needed in order to apply to CRNA programs. There are some programs that accept experience outside of ICU.

Q: Can I be a traveling CRNA?
A: Yes. The technical term for this is an independent contractor, informally called a "1099 employee", freelancer, or locum CRNA. There are recruitment agencies that facilitate contracts between medical facilities and CRNAs for these types of positions. Sometimes, you can also connect directly with the facility to be contracted for your anesthesia services, cutting out the middleman. Contracts can vary in time from one day to an indefinite period. If you have a permanent residency, there is a time limit you can travel without being penalized. It is recommended that you discuss this with your tax preparer. As a freelancer, you will need to be provided a higher hourly pay rate since you will cover your malpractice insurance, self-employment taxes, retirement contributions, health coverage, and disability insurance on your own. Currently, the average salary for a full-time traveling CRNA is about $220,000.

Q: Do I need to have my own business to work freelance?
A: No, you don't have to. Where you live and what you would like to do business-wise will help determine whether or not you should incorporate. For instance, if you plan on staying within your state and only do contract work in that area, you may want to form an LLC (limited liability company) over an S corporation. LLC is state-

specific. You can elect to have your LLC taxed as an S corporation, avoiding the 15.3% self-employment taxes on distributions or draws. If you create an LLC, you are technically an "employee" of your business and must pay yourself a reasonable salary, as shown on a W-2 tax form. If you only plan on working a few shifts per year as an independent contractor, then forming an S corporation or LLC may not be financially beneficial. I am not a CPA nor an attorney, so I suggest speaking to a professional in those areas about forming your business plan and gathering further information to make the right decision for you.

Q: What are the differences between CRNA, AA, and Anesthesiologist?
A: An AA or anesthesiology assistant holds a master's degree with a concentration in anesthesia. An AA is to an anesthesiologist what a physician assistant is to a licensed physician. AAs are not licensed to practice in every state; only fifteen states currently allow it. An AA must work under the license and direction of an anesthesiologist. Anesthesiologists are medical doctors or doctors of osteopathy who have graduated from medical school, completed a residency in anesthesia, and sometimes an additional fellowship in a subspecialty like pain management, pediatrics, or cardiothoracic anesthesiology. For more information on CRNAs, see chapter one.

Q: I heard that anesthesiologists hate CRNAs. Is there any truth to that?
A: I don't know about people hating others in each profession, but the politics of anesthesia have been a growing concern for over sixty years. The AANA and ASA (American Society of Anesthesiologists) have yet to come to a compromise about nurse anesthetists working autonomously in all fifty states. There is also the issue of CRNAs being able to bill for services without an

anesthesiologist's supervision. There have been strides made for CRNAs and anesthesiologists to come to a common agreement. Our training is different but not inferior to that of anesthesiologists, and I believe we should be allowed to practice independently to the full scope that we have been trained. I enjoy a collaborative team approach when giving anesthesia and believe there are enough jobs, opportunities, and patients out there for all of us to practice successfully. One of my biggest pet peeves is when some anesthesiologists, specifically those who think nurse anesthetists are unsafe and unqualified to give quality care, make such judgmental remarks while sitting in another room. I have no personal issue with anesthesiologists, but downplaying and slandering CRNAs as dangerous and incompetent is not only derogatory - it is untrue and disrespectful. There is no published data stating that care provided by an anesthesiologist is better than that of a CRNA. I believe it's time for the public to be educated on what really goes on in the operating room and who is at the head of the bed for over 45,000,000 anesthetics each year – The CRNAs.

Q: How do you handle working with difficult people?
A: There are a number of personalities in the surgical team setting. Dealing with nurses, surgeons, techs, anesthesiologists, and other nurse anesthetists can be stressful and overwhelming. The best advice I can give you is to go in everyday with a positive attitude, ready to learn as much as you possibly can. Introduce yourself to everyone and follow the instructions given to you by the more seasoned professionals. You know how to deal with difficult patients because you've done it as a nurse in the ICU. Don't forget that the most important person in the room during surgery is the patient and you are his or her advocate. You will be paying a lot of your money to learn and understand how to become a CRNA. At the end of the

day, remember that is your goal! Don't forget that. Humble yourself and get through it.

Q: Why do you call yourself a nurse anesthesiologist?
A: According to the New Oxford American Dictionary, the suffix "-ologist" simply means, "a subject of study; a branch of knowledge." Nurse anesthesiologists have studied and trained in the field of anesthesia. Read more about the history and terminology of the profession in chapter one.

Q: Am I ready to apply to CRNA school?
A: Only you know the answer to that. Don't let anyone else tell you otherwise, especially if he or she is not a CRNA. Once you have your level one trauma ICU experience and have completed all of the other necessary requirements to apply, then go for it! You won't know the answer until you do it. Read more about the CRNA application and supplemental materials in chapter three.

Q: In which states can I practice independently as a CRNA?
A: To date, you can practice independently without anesthesiologist supervision in any of the following seventeen states that have opted out of the federal physician supervision requirement: Iowa, Nebraska, Idaho, Minnesota, New Hampshire, New Mexico, Kansas, North Dakota, Washington, Alaska, Oregon, Montana, South Dakota, Wisconsin, California, Colorado, and Kentucky.

Common Acronyms in Nurse Anesthesiology

- AANA- American Association of Nurse Anesthetist
- ASA- American Society of Anesthesiologists
- CRNA- Certified Registered Nurse Anesthetist or Anesthesiologist

- APRN- Advance Practice Registered Nurse
- NP- Nurse Practitioner
- SRNA- Student Registered Nurse Anesthetist
- RN- Registered Nurse
- LPN- License Practical Nurse
- CNA- Certified Nursing Assistant
- MD- Medical Doctor
- DO-Doctor of Osteopathy
- MDA- Medical Doctor of Anesthesia
- PA- Physician Assistant
- AA- Anesthesiologist Assistant
- GRE- Graduate Record Examination
- CCRN- Critical Care Registered Nurse
- AACN- American Association of Critical Care Nurses
- ACLS- Advance Cardiac Life Support
- PALS- Pediatric Advanced Life Support
- BLS- Basic Life support/ CPR
- ICU- Intensive Care Unit
- IABP- intra-aortic balloon pump
- ECMO- Extracorporeal membrane oxygenation
- EKG- electrocardiograph
- ABG- Arterial Blood Gas

Bibliography

All CRNA Schools. "The Cost of Nurse Anesthetist School."

Accessed on February 1, 2019.

http://www.all-crna-schools.com/schools-by-cost/

American Association of Critical-Care Nurses. "Initial Eligibiliy

Requirements & Fees." Accessed March 17, 2019.

https://www.aacn.org/certification/get-certified/ccrn-adult

American Association of Nurse Anesthetists. "CRNA Fact Sheet."

Last modified February 28.

https://www.aana.com/membership/become-a-crna/crna-fact-

sheet

Diversity in Nurse Anesthesia Mentorship Program. Accessed on

February 1, 2019. https://diversitycrna.org

Finnamore, Hoyt. "Celebrating Nurse Anesthetist Education – Alice

Magaw (1860-1928): Mother of Anesthesia." *Sharing Mayo*

Clinic. January 26, 2015.

https://sharing.mayoclinic.org/2015/01/26/celebrating-nurse-

anesthetist-education-alice-magaw-1860-1928-mother-of-
anesthesia/

National Board for Certification & Recertification of Nurse
Anesthetists. "NCE FAQ."
https://www.nbcrna.com/exams/nce-resources/nce-faq. Last
modified August 1, 2016.

Stewart, Angie. "The Joint Commission addresses the OR
temperature standard – 4 details." *Becker's ASC Review.*
February 16, 2018. https://www.beckersasc.com/asc-
accreditation-and-patient-safety/the-joint-commission-
addresses-or-temperature-standard-4-details.html

U.S. News and World Report. "What is a Nurse Anesthetist?"
Accessed March 17, 2019.
https://money.usnews.com/careers/best-jobs/nurse-
anesthetist

About the Author

Crystal Grant is a Certified Registered Nurse Anesthetist and a graduate of UMDNJ, currently Rutgers University-Newark. She lives in Western Massachusetts with her two dogs, Ryder the Morkie and Teddy the Bichon. In her free time, Crystal enjoys spending time with her family, writing, reading, traveling to the Caribbean, and shopping. She currently does frequent CRNA trivia giveaways and enjoys teaching and helping others who are interested in pursuing a career in health care.

Follow Crystal on Instagram @thesixfigureCRNA and @crysgcrna

For contact information and to request Crystal for speaking engagements, send an email to thesixfigureCRNA@gmail.com.

Thank you to all who helped me achieve this goal. It's been a long road, but we made it! CRNA photos provided by:

Randy Barnard
Dr. Deborah Greer
Ebony Page
Capt. James Winters II
Joanne Hill
Florence Zilko
Jaclyn H
Deji Babaloa
Junior Senat
Darolyn Milburn
LaTonya Mims
JoAnn Nava
Sarah Schilling
Marquetta Butler
Rose Vernot
Donnell Carter

The Editor:
This book was edited by Brittany J. McKeldin.
Contact Brittany for your project via email at
bjmckeldin@gmail.com.

Stay Tuned for future works from the author, including:
The Six Figure Movement
The Super CRNA comic series
The guide to 1099

Made in the USA
Middletown, DE
24 December 2019

81765872R00040